"How I Conquered DIABETES"

Bruce Gould

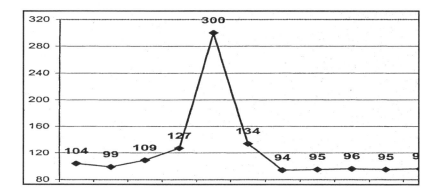

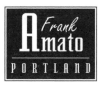

Frank Amato
PORTLAND

The material you are about to read is not medical advice. It is not intended as medical advice. It is not a substitute for medical advice. In every case, one seeking medical advice should seek out and talk to a licensed physician. A physician is the person best able to counsel and advise persons in the area of medical needs. Medical decisions should not be made by any person without first consulting with a physician. Likewise, it may be wise to speak to a physician before making any decisions that relate to your health. Discuss with your physician any medical conditions you may have as well as any medicines you may be taking to treat such conditions. If you are taking vitamin supplements, you should also advise your treating physician of the same. This is especially true and important for persons diagnosed as diabetics, who are on dialysis, who are pregnant or nursing or who may be taking diabetes medicines or diuretics or medicines of any kind. In all cases, proceed carefully and only under a doctor's care. To repeat, the material you have just read in the previous 90+ pages is not medical advice. It is not intended as medical advice. It is not a substitute for medical advice. In every case, one seeking medical advice should seek out and talk to a licensed physician.

Published in 2006 by
Frank Amato Publications, Inc.
P.O. Box 82112
Portland, Oregon 97282
(503) 653-8108
©2003 Bruce Gould
www.amatobooks.com

Softbound ISBN: 1-57188-381-9 • Softbound UPC: 0-81127-00215-3

Printed in Hong Kong

1 3 5 7 9 10 8 6 4 2

My name is Bruce Gould and this is my story. It may be helpful to you or to someone you know or someone you love. My story may even save the life of yourself, someone you know, or that someone you love. If it does, it will be well worth the effort I am putting into telling you about my situation. I am hopeful that you, or that someone you know, or that someone you love, will benefit by this report.

I was born in the small town of Okanogan, Washington, a town with a population of about 2,000 very nice people. I grew up here, went to the local schools for twelve years, moved away to attend college and then came back home in order that my children might also grow up in a small town. For most of the years of my life, I had no reason to suspect there were any major problems with respect to my health and I generally considered myself a healthy person. Up until the year 1996, I had regular medical checkups every few years and, in the year 1996, my personal medical records provided me with blood sugar numbers, cholesterol numbers, LDL cholesterol numbers, HDL cholesterol numbers and my triglyceride levels. Graphs of my 1988-1996 medical records showing each of these categories are reproduced on the following pages.

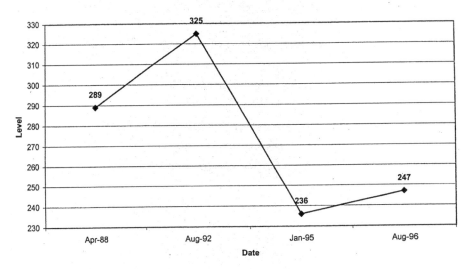

Total Cholesterol
April 1988 - August 1996

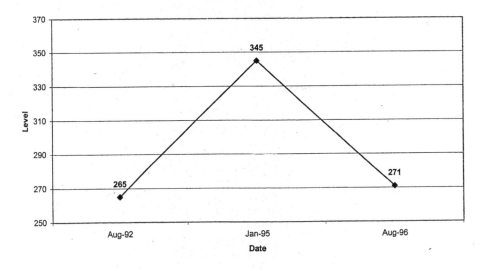

Triglycerides
August 1992 - August 1996

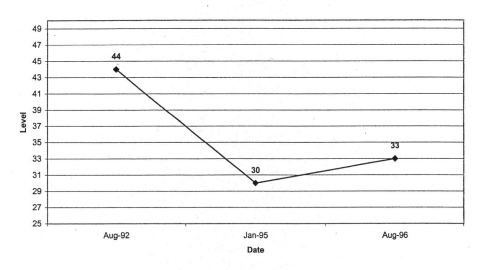

Cholesterol - HDL
August 1992 - August 1996

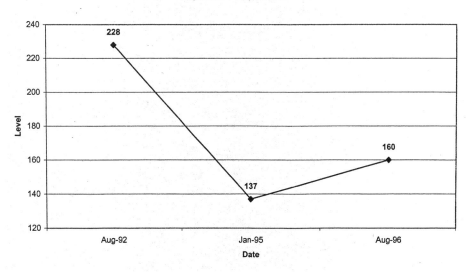

Cholesterol - LDL
August 1992 - August 1996

5

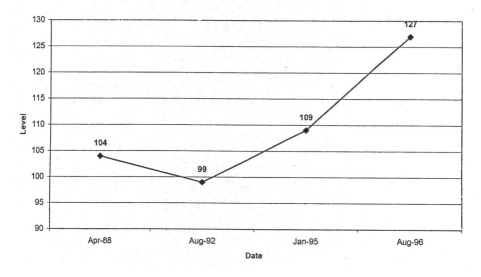

Blood Sugar
April 1988 - August 1996

Any interested person can go to any medical reference book at his or her local library and read all about blood sugar, cholesterol, HDL cholesterol, LDL cholesterol and triglycerides. The medical literature basically tells the reader that blood sugar is the amount of sugar circulating in one's blood at any given time, cholesterol is a fatty substance known as a lipid which is essential for life. The medical literature will tell you that the liver in one's body generally produces most of the cholesterol a person needs and that this cholesterol may be broken down into many parts, two of which are LDL cholesterol, also known as low density lipoprotein, and HDL cholesterol, known as high

6

density lipoprotein. In today's medical literature, it is often stressed that the good cholesterol is the HDL cholesterol and the bad cholesterol is the LDL cholesterol. Ratios are often computed to determine the relationship between how much HDL one has relative to how much LDL and how much HDL one has relative to total cholesterol in a person's body at any given time.

When reading the medical literature, you may read that triglycerides is also a medical term for certain lipids or fats circulating in one's blood. It is said that triglyceride molecules have a different chemical structure from cholesterol molecules. In 1996, when my body was producing the kind of numbers that are represented by the graphs on pages 4, 5, and 6, I knew almost nothing about the entire subject of blood sugars, cholesterol, HDL cholesterol, LDL cholesterol and triglycerides. I did know that in 1996 I felt relatively good and didn't feel I had any major health worries. I lived life in a normal fashion eating what I thought was a normal diet. I moved through life as though catastrophe would never strike. I was ignorant and I was innocent and, in less than seven years, my ignorance would disappear and my innocence would vanish. Here is how this change to my life came about.

By 2003, I was tired all the time. A general fatigue seemed to have settled into my body. I also seemed to have to go to the bathroom numerous times during the night, which was a change from my 1996 bathroom habits. I often felt dehydrated and thirsty. In addition, there was a definite eye pressure that was bothering me, especially the pressure behind my right eye. My vision seemed to be blurred and I also noted that I was having more headaches than usual. There was a general numbness in my toes that produced a sensation similar to having parts of my feet asleep all the time. By January of 2003, I knew that something was not right with respect to my body. It did not make sense to me that I should be so tired so much of the time, including a general tiredness during my work day. By January of 2003, if my two children proposed a fishing or vacation trip, I had to consider whether I had the stamina to undertake such a venture before giving them a "yes" or "no" answer. This had not been the situation back in 1996 when my body was producing the medical numbers shown on pages 4, 5 and 6. What was happening in 2003 that was so different? I knew that something was wrong with me and so I scheduled an appointment with a family physician and this is what I discovered.

My catastrophe was about to strike.

January 2003 blood sugar graph

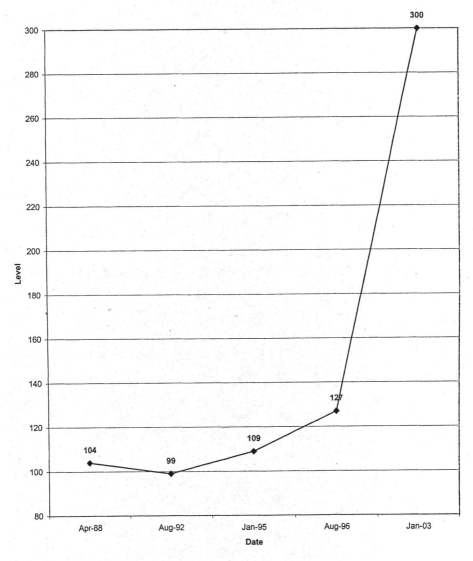

Blood Sugar
April 1988 - January 2003

Somehow in time period from August of 1996 until January 22nd of 2003, my blood sugars had risen from 127 to 300. How did this happen? I attribute it to my innocence and my ignorance and the action and non-action taken by me due to my lack of knowledge.

A rise in blood sugar levels from 127 to 300 is a catastrophic rise for the amount of sugar circulating in one's body. In today's medical literature, it is often stated that one has type 2 "diabetes" when fasting plasma glucose (FPG) passes 126mg/dl. My January 2003 fasting plasma glucose was 300mg/dl.

In 1996, with a fasting plasma glucose level of 127mg/dl, I was just entering into a seven-year period of undiagnosed diabetes. By 2003, when I found out what had happened, **I had been a type 2 diabetic for seven years without even knowing it.** No wonder I was always tired, dehydrated, urinating frequently, with pressure on my eyes and my feet feeling numb. Take a good look at my January 2003 blood sugar graph on page 9 again. This graph represents seven years of my innocence and ignorance – it represents seven years of lived with but undiagnosed type 2 diabetes. The victim of seven years of the medical disease known as type 2 diabetes **was me.**

Who do I blame for allowing this "type 2 diabetes" to exist in my body for these seven long years without my knowledge of the same? I blame myself. Now that I am no longer innocent and ignorant, reading the medical literature I can quickly see that the major symptoms of type 2 diabetes are:

1. A frequent desire to urinate.
2. An unusual thirst.
3. Blurred vision.
4. A feeling of being tired most of the time for no apparent reason.
5. Leg pain
6. Nerve damage
7. Poor circulation.

I had at least five of these symptoms, possibly six. In my innocence and ignorance I did not know that I was just one in a long line of "undiagnosed type 2 diabetics" in the world. It is said that there are about 16,000,000 Americans who have diabetes, six percent of the population. It was estimated in 1999 that 5-6 million people in America have type 2 diabetes and don't even know it. In 1999, I was one of those 5-6 million. The fact that so many people have type 2 diabetes, without knowledge of the same, has led researchers to refer to this disease as the **"silent killer"**. By the time many of these 5-6 million people learn they are "diabetic" they will already be at a point where they face serious risk of suffering a major health illness.

After I had my medical checkup in 1996, I continued eating in my normal fashion and my weight gradually increased. With each year of one's life, activities often diminish and weight often advances. The normal weight for someone of my height is about 175 pounds. At my peak, in the years between 1996 and 2003, I was probably 30 pounds overweight. For many type 2 diabetics, excess weight goes hand in hand with the diabetic condition. The medical literature tells us that people who are significantly overweight have a far greater chance of becoming diabetic than thin or normal weight people. If a person is overweight, regular medical checkups with a family physician are advisable so that there is not a progression from excess weight to diabetes. It is very important for overweight people to keep in regular contact with their physician so that this road to the disease of diabetes can be avoided.

Diabetes is not a benign medical condition. The consequences of maintaining high blood sugar levels, such as my 300mg/dl, for several years are very serious. Medical literature tells us that type 2 diabetes is a **serious life-threatening disease**.

1. The medical literature tells us that diabetes is a leading cause of **kidney failure**. Many people who require long-term kidney dialysis require this treatment because they have the disease of diabetes.
2. The medical literature tells us that diabetes is a leading cause of **blindness**. Cataracts, glaucoma, retinopathy are all diseases of the eyes and all these diseases are sometimes found in the eyes of people who have diabetes.
3. The medical literature tells us that diabetes is a major cause of **nerve disease or neuropathy**. I know this from personal experience. When my toes and feet felt like they were asleep, I was experiencing the neuropathy caused by my seven years of undiagnosed type 2 diabetes.
4. The medical literature tells us that **coronary artery disease** is the most common reason for death in type 2 diabetics. It is written that 20% of all people with diabetes die of heart attacks. The death rate from heart attacks for diabetics is more than twice the death rate for non-diabetics.
5. The medical literature tells us that more than 50,000-foot amputations occur in the United States each year and that half of them are done on people with diabetes. Diabetes is the leading cause of **limb amputation** in America.

On January 22nd, 2003, when I learned that I had type 2 diabetes and had probably suffered from this disease for the previous seven years was I scared? **You bet I was scared. I was really scared.**

With my blood sugars rising from 127mg/dl to 300mg/dl, I not only had type 2 diabetes, I had a very bad case of type 2 diabetes. Faced with the very real possibility of **coronary heart disease**, **blindness**, **kidney failure**, **neuropathy** and **limb amputation**, I was really scared. I realized both that I didn't have much of a fun future to look forward to and that I had every good reason for doing everything I could to avoid the medical consequences of my seven years of undiagnosed type 2 diabetes.

It is my personal opinion, and this is not based on any medical diagnosis, conversation, or prediction, that had I known as much about type 2 "diabetes" in 1996 as I know about type 2 diabetes today, I would never have gotten type 2 "diabetes" in the first place. It is my personal opinion that I could have avoided this disease of diabetes entirely, starting back in 1996, if I had only known then what I know now. There is no way to prove this, but I am personally 100% convinced that such is the case.

I decided that to solve my difficult medical problem, I needed to **seek a solution.** "Solution seeking" now became my personal objective. I wanted to try, in my limited way, to overcome seven years of innocence and ignorance and to try to return myself to the best possible health that I could return myself to knowing that I had been suffering an undiagnosed disease for seven years.

The primary thing I knew in January of 2003 was that I had to **immediately** reduce the sugars or glucose in my blood stream. This was absolutely essential. If I were not able to reduce the sugar solution circulating in my blood then **coronary artery disease**, **kidney disease**, **blindness**, **neuropathy** and possible **limb amputation** would be my future life. In January of 2003, it appeared to me as a reasonably intelligent person, that there were three paths I could go down seeking a solution to my disease.

I could, working with my physician, commence insulin shots immediately, commencing within twenty-four hours of January 22, 2003.

I could, working with my physician, commence drug treatment immediately, commencing within twenty-four hours of January 22, 2003.

Or I could, working partly with my physician and partly on my own initiative, come up with a solution that would serve to control my tendency to be overweight, my high cholesterol levels and my type 2 diabetic disease.

This I knew for sure, I didn't want to have a **heart attack** brought on by my diabetic condition. I didn't want **to go blind** because of my diabetic condition. I knew that I didn't want **my kidneys to fail** due to my diabetic disease. Finally, all the limbs I had-I wanted to keep. I didn't want any **limb amputation** caused directly or indirectly by the disease known as diabetes. I could live with a little neuropathy in my toes, but I didn't want to die, I didn't want my kidneys to fail, I didn't want to go blind and I didn't want any limbs amputated. To avoid these perils, I started to reduce the sugar or glucose in my blood. To cause this reduction, I realized I could do either or both of the following,

> Make a change in the food I was eating.
> Start using pharmaceutical drugs.

I personally ruled out taking insulin as an alternative. I would select insulin as a last resort, if and only if there was no other possible method for me to return my body to a reasonable state of health. With insulin removed from the table of alternatives this left a choice between changing my food habits and using drugs. I could try one approach, or the other, or a combination of the two.

I am a great admirer and a very cautious person when it comes to using pharmaceutical drugs. I think I read somewhere that in the year 1900, the average life span of an American was 45 years. Today, a person lives to be 75 or more, on the average. This 30-year increase in life span in less than one hundred years is connected in many ways to the real health benefits offered to humans by pharmaceutical drugs. I believe in pharmaceutical drugs; I also just happen to be a very cautious person. If possible, I would prefer to live my life taking as few pharmaceutical drugs as possible. This seems to make sense to me. Every so often, once in a while, now and then, a person will read in the newspaper about a serious problem apparently or allegedly caused by the use of a pharmaceutical drug.

*Morris Plains, N. J. March 21, 2000 – Warner-Lambert Company announced today that it is voluntarily discontinuing the sale of REZULIN (TROGLITAZONE) Tablets, **its therapy for the treatment of type 2 diabetes**, although the Company continues to believe that the benefits of the drug outweigh its associated risks.*

Patients taking REZULIN should consult with their physicians as soon as possible to discuss alternative therapies. Warner-Lambert will work closely with the Food and Drug Administration and other constituencies to assure a safe and efficient transition for patients as they switch to alternative therapies.

The Company has always believed that it is essential for patients and physicians to receive accurate and objective information regarding the benefits and risks of REZULIN. It was for this reason that Warner-Lambert requested a public meeting of the FDA's expert Advisory Committee. However, repeated media reports sensationalizing the risks associated with REZULIN have created an environment in which patients and physicians are simply unable to make well-informed decisions regarding the safety and efficacy of REZULIN. Under these circumstances, and after discussions this evening with the FDA, we have decided it is in the best interests of patients to discontinue marketing REZULIN at this time.

This was the press release by the Warner-Lambert Company. On that same day, the US Dept Health & Human Services issued their FDA release with respect to REZULIN.

P00-8
FOR IMMEDIATE RELEASE
March 21, 2000

FOOD AND DRUG ADMINISTRATION
Print Media: 301-827-6242
Broadcast Media: 301-827-3434
Consumer Inquiries:888-INFO-FDA

REZULIN TO BE WITHDRAWN FROM THE MARKET

FDA today asked the manufacturer of Rezulin (troglitazone) -- a drug used to treat type 2 diabetes mellitus-- to remove the product from the market. The drug's manufacturer, Parke-Davis/Warner-Lambert, has agreed to FDA's request.

FDA took this action after its review of recent safety data on Rezulin and two similar drugs, rosiglitazone (Avandia) and pioglitazone (Actos), showed that Rezulin is more toxic to the liver than the other two drugs. Data to date show that Avandia and Actos, both approved in the past year, offer the same benefits as Rezulin without the same risk.

"When considered as a whole, the pre-marketing clinical data and post-marketing safety data from Rezulin as compared to similar, alternative diabetes drugs indicate that continued use of Rezulin now poses an unacceptable risk to patients," said Dr. Janet Woodcock, Director of FDA's Center for Drug Evaluation and Research. "We are now confident that patients have safer alternatives in this important class of diabetes drugs," she added.

Severe liver toxicity has been known to occur with Rezulin since 1997. In consultation with FDA, Parke-Davis has strengthened the drug's labeling several times and has recommended close monitoring of liver function in patients taking Rezulin.

In March 1999, FDA's Endocrine and Metabolic Drugs Advisory Committee reviewed the status of Rezulin and its risk of liver toxicity and recommended continued availability of this drug in a select group of patients -- patients not well-controlled on other diabetes drugs.

Since then, FDA has continued to actively monitor adverse events associated with Rezulin, as well as Avandia and Actos. After up to nine months of marketing experience with these two newer drugs, it has now become clear that these newer drugs have less risk of severe liver toxicity than Rezulin.

Patients using Rezulin are urged to contact their physicians for information about alternative treatments. Patients should not discontinue taking Rezulin or other treatments for diabetes without discussing alternative therapies with their physicians.

For more information about Rezulin, go to FDA's MedWatch site.

19

If you go to the internet and do some research on the pharmaceutical drug "Rezulin" you will undoubtedly find numerous law firms advising prospective clients about "Rezulin". If you read some of the web site statements made (and I am personally unable to guarantee the accuracy of any statements made on the internet by anyone but myself) you will find comments like these:

1. On January 29, 1997, the FDA approved Rezulin for the treatment of type 2 diabetes.
2. Rezulin was withdrawn from the market on March 21, 2000 after several deaths had been recorded for patients using Rezulin.
3. Dr. Grahm, the FDA's leading specialist in evaluating and preventing deaths caused by prescription drugs, is reported to have estimated that one out of every 1,800 Rezulin patients could be expected to suffer health problems.
4. Patients with moderately elevated ALT levels at the start of drug therapy should not be initiated on Rezulin.
5. Patients taking the type 2 diabetes drug Rezulin (troglitazone) should be monitored frequently for signs of injury to the liver.
6. The drug Rezulin, designed to stabilize blood sugar levels in type 2 diabetic patients, could

be the next big wave of pharmaceutical litigation, plaintiff's attorneys nationwide predict.

Notice item number one. On January 29, 1997, the FDA approved Rezulin for the treatment of type 2 diabetes. **Now remember my history.** In 1996, I had a blood sugar test and it registered 127mg/dl. Today a fasting blood sugar level of 127mg/dl is an indication of type 2 diabetes disease. Had my physician, in the month of February, 1997, prescribed Rezulin for me it is quite possible that I might have been one of those using Rezulin who suffered liver failure or even death. Thus, as bad as it seems, the fact that I probably suffered from undiagnosed type 2 diabetes disease for the seven years from 1996 until 2003, may have been a blessing in disguise. Had my diabetic disease been diagnosed during the time period that Rezulin was available, I might well be dead today. Perhaps, in an odd sort of way, it is a good thing my diabetic condition was not diagnosed during the time period that Rezulin was available to treat it.

In January of 2003, when I was diagnosed a diabetic, I faced three choices of treatment (1) insulin (2) drugs or (3) a third alternative that I could come up with on my own using my own intelligence and research abilities.

Let me tell you what I know about insulin. I know

almost nothing about insulin. The little I know about insulin is that for people who need insulin to stay alive, it is a very beneficial aid. If I needed insulin to stay alive, I would be taking insulin right now. But when I examined the literature and read that many type 2 diabetics do not need insulin to stay alive, I avoided this alternative for my blood sugar control.

In January of 2003, the issue of blood sugar and how to reduce it became the **critical issue of my life.** If insulin was removed as a necessary alternative, then the medical literature told me that there were three methods of reducing the amount of sugar in my blood,

1. By taking pharmaceutical drugs to control my blood sugars, or
2. By using good food practices to control my blood sugars, or
3. A combination of (1) and (2).

Quite frankly, I was afraid of depending on drugs. I didn't want to fall victim to a Rezulin type drug and lose my liver and possibly my life. Were I to be given the choice of whether I wanted to be tired all the time, urinating frequently at night, suffering pressure behind my eyes and facing coronary heart disease, blindness, kidney failure and limb amputation somewhere down the road or losing my liver because I was taking a pharmaceutical drug that destroyed my liver in a matter of days or weeks or even months, I wouldn't have to think about the choices very long. I didn't want to take insulin and I didn't want to be committed to a lifetime of taking pharmaceutical drugs, so what was I to do?

Eating Sugars

Medical literature tells us that if one drinks alcohol, alcohol will enter the blood stream. Medical literature also tells us that if one eats sugars, sugars will enter the blood stream. It is written that once sugar is in the blood stream, excess sugars can sometimes be removed or more efficiently used by the body through the usage of pharmaceutical drugs. Another way to reduce excess sugars in the blood stream, it appeared to me after reading the medical literature, is not to consume large quantities of sugar in the first place. Once I was no longer innocent and ignorant and had a vague idea as to what was going on in my own body, it seemed to me that for me to eat excess sugars was a bit like throwing mud on my car. I could throw a lot of mud and sand and gravel on my car and then try to find a nice polish or wax that would try to remove this muddy dirty mess without scratching my car's surface, or I could simply not throw mud, sand and gravel on my car in the first place. The choice, for me, then became,

1. Should I throw lots of mud on my car and then try to remove it, or
2. Should I not throw much mud on my car in the first place so that I would not have to remove it?

I selected the second choice. It was, for me a matter of common sense. For me, eating an excess amount of sugars became identified in my mind with throwing lots of sand and gravel and mud on a new bright shinny car.

I kept eating food, but I **immediately** reduced my sugar intake.

(Here is what I started to eat – see next page)

List "A" - Foods I eat.

©Bruce Gould, 2003

Sunflower Seeds
Turkey
Blueberries
Chicken
Tuna Fish
Celery
Salmon
Olives
Cottage Cheese
Steaks
Cabbage
Broccoli
Cauliflower
Asparagus
Turkey Hotdogs
Avocado
Hamburger Patties
Onions
Garlic
Cream
Mustard
Spinach
Lettuce
Cucumbers
Small Quantities Of Fruit

List "A" - Foods I eat.

Mayonnaise
Hollandaise Sauce
Beef & Pork & Turkey Bologna
Butter
Cinnamon
Blue Cheese
Feta Cheese
Swiss Cheese
Dijon Mustard
Horseradish
Corn Oil
Olive Oil
Lamb
Bacon
Pork Loin
Pork Sausage
Pork Spareribs
Pork Tenderloin
Beef Broth
Fish Of Almost Every Kind
Chili Pepper
Small Quantities Of Peanuts
Mushrooms
Other Poultry Of Almost Every Kind
Other Meats Of Almost Every Kind

List "B" - Foods I do not eat

©Bruce Gould, 2003

Bananas
Cake
Cookies
Sugar
Spaghetti
Potatoes
Bread
Breakfast Cereal
Beans
Ice Cream
Hamburger & Hotdog Buns
Crackers
Raisins
Milk
Catsup
Honey
Dried Fruit
Fruit Juices
Flour
Corn
Candy
Potato Chips
Oranges
Cherries
Carrots

List "B" - Foods I do not eat

©Bruce Gould, 2003

Rice
Grapes
Pizza
Most Soups
Yogurt
Grapefruit
Ginger Snaps
English Muffins
Pineapple
French Fries
Soft Drinks
Casseroles
Pretzels
Pie
Cocoa
Pudding
Cranberry Sauce
Syrup
Muffins
Lifesavers
Spaghetti Sauce
Oysters
Sweet Potatoes
Sweet And Sour Sauce
Chocolate Milk

How I make my decisions as to what foods I will or will not eat.

Once I had read the medical literature and was no longer innocent and ignorant, I learned that the word carbohydrate is really just another word for a form of sugar. I realized that during the seven years from 1996 until 2003, when I was eating a large amount of carbohydrates daily, I was actually **eating a large quantity of sugar daily.** Since I now connected eating large quantities of carbohydrates with eating large quantities of sugar, it appeared to me that the common sense thing to do was to reduce the amount of carbohydrates and sugar that I put into my body each day to see what happened to my blood sugar levels. I also wanted to know what effect this would have on my cholesterol level and my weight.

In my innocence and ignorance, I never thought that eating a baked potato could be compared with eating a candy bar. However, once I read in the medical literature that after it enters one's blood stream, most starch is broken down into a form of sugar, eating starch became pretty much like eating candy bars to me. I had also never considered milk to contain a form of sugar, but it does, even skim milk. I knew ice cream contained sugar, but carrots? Could a slice of bread or a hamburger bun be seen as a form of sugar? The answer is yes, in the sense that the starch or carbohydrates in a bread product will, in the end, be reduced to a sugar-like substance circulating in the blood stream.

One of the first things I did in January of 2003 was purchase a **"blood sugar monitor".** A blood sugar monitor is a little like an air pressure gage used to check the air pressure in one's automobile tires. If you want to know the air pressure in your car's tire, you put a gage over the valve and come up with a number. If you want to know how much sugar is circulating in your blood at any given time, the medical literature tells us either to see your family physician or use a home blood sugar monitor. Put a small drop of your blood on the strip in the monitor and a number will pop up. In 1996, the number for the sugar in my blood had been 127mg/dl. Seven years later, on January 22nd, 2003, the number was 300mg/dl. At 127 mg/dl a person is designated as a type 2 diabetic. At 300 mg/dl a person is designated as a type 2 diabetic in very bad condition. Finding a blood sugar reading of 300mg/dl is like testing the air pressure in your car's tire expecting a reading of 28psi and coming up with a reading of 100psi. **This is definitely not good news.**

So, by now I had read the medical literature, learned what sugar was and what carbohydrates were, how the two were similar in many ways and I got myself a home blood monitor for about $90. I figured the $90 investment was well worth the cost to turn myself from an innocent and ignorant type 2 diabetic into an informed and knowledge-able type 2 diabetic. If I could prevent a future life of blindness, amputation of limbs, coronary artery disease, kidney disease, excess weight and possi-bly high cholesterol, the $90 would be the best $90 I ever spent. I then started to use the blood sugar monitor on a regular basis, monitoring my blood sugar several times a day to see if my new food habits would help to lower my blood sugars and to keep them low. **In essence, here is what I did,**

1. I started to read the ingredient label on every food I ate. If the food did not have a label on it, I looked that food up in a reference book to see what the food was composed of.
2. If the food contained lots of carbohydrates (meaning lots of grams of sugar for me) I did not eat that food.
3. If the food contained few carbohydrates (meaning not much sugar for me) I would consider eating that food.

4. I monitored my blood sugar levels on my $90 home monitor several times a day.
5. If I noticed my circulating blood sugar levels advancing and remaining high after eating certain foods, I did not eat those foods again.
6. If I noticed my blood sugar levels remaining steady or declining several hours after eating certain foods, I added those foods to my preferred list.
7. During this time, I was consuming mainly low to moderately low carbohydrate foods that I had found listed in the medical literature. Within the course of 30 days, I gradually developed a list of foods that I would eat and a list of foods that I would not eat. These lists are reproduced above.

My guideline is very simple: **I will eat anything that is not poison which helps to keep my blood sugar, cholesterol and weight levels low, always striving to keep my blood sugar below 127mg/dl based on a pre-breakfast reading.**

I will not eat anything that results in consistent high blood sugar, cholesterol or weight levels for me or causes my blood sugar levels to register at 127mg/dl or higher based on a pre-breakfast reading after not eating during the nighttime.

This is a pretty simple rule. I can eat anything that helps to keep my circulating blood sugar, weight and cholesterol levels low and I won't eat anything that keeps any of these levels high. I consider that every food, beverage and fruit is on the table. What I decide to eat depends on what my blood sugar monitor tells me after I have eaten a particular food.

What was the result of the program I adopted for myself? Let's look at blood sugar levels first, then we will look at cholesterol levels and weight levels.

I started to monitor my blood sugar on January 22nd, 2003. The attached record is from January through March of 2003. This is what my home blood sugar monitoring shows for those 60 days. The starting point was a blood sugar reading taken at my doctor's office on January 22nd, 2003. It showed a level of 300 mg/dl. On January 23rd, 2003, I had my blood sugar level re-tested by a different doctor (always get a second opinion, remember). The January 23rd level was 298 mg/dl. On January 24th, my blood sugar was checked in the office of a diabetic nurse. The reading was 239 mg/dl. All of the other readings were done on my home blood sugar monitor. The results are reproduced on the following pages.

Home Blood Sugar Reading – Week of Jan 19th –26th 2003

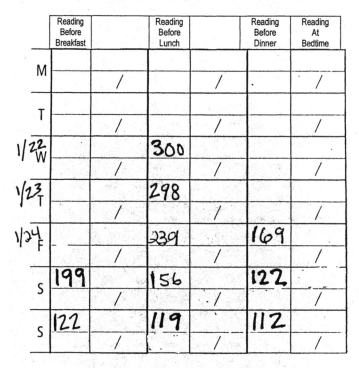

	Reading Before Breakfast		Reading Before Lunch		Reading Before Dinner	Reading At Bedtime
M		/		/	.	/
T		/		/		/
1/22 W		/	300	/		/
1/23 T		/	298	/		/
1/24 F		/	239	/	169	/
S	199	/	156	/	122	/
S	122	/	119	/	112	/

Home Blood Sugar Reading – Week of Jan 27th - Feb 2nd 2003

	Reading Before Breakfast		Reading Before Lunch		Reading Before Dinner	Reading At Bedtime
M	113	/	123	/	89	141
T	107	/	77	/	77	128
W	120	/	86	/	93	124
T	115	/	84	/	107	110
F	118	/	94	/	97	105
S	117	/	82	/	102	129
S	98	/	79	/	94	136

Home Blood Sugar Reading – Week of Feb 3rd - 9th 2003

	Reading Before Breakfast		Reading Before Lunch		Reading Before Dinner	Reading At Bedtime
M	123		111		86	92
		/		/		/
T	109		100		92	119
		/		/		/
W	113		91		96	94
		/		/		/
T	106		102		99	109
		/		/		/
F	120		113		98	110
		/		/		/
S	121		97		99	106
		/		/		/
S	123		98		101	109
		/		/		/

Home Blood Sugar Reading – Week of Feb 10th – 16th 2003

	Reading Before Breakfast		Reading Before Lunch		Reading Before Dinner	Reading At Bedtime
M	109		112		96	95
		/		/		/
T	118		81		90	97
		/		/		/
W	116		96		98	101
		/		/		/
T	107		113		99	98
		/		/		/
F	100		99		88	99
		/		/		/
S	107		113		102	106
		/		/		/
S	112		106		97	95
		/		/		/

Home Blood Sugar Reading – Week of Feb 17th –23rd 2003

	Reading Before Breakfast		Reading Before Lunch		Reading Before Dinner	Reading At Bedtime
M	108	/	108	/	91	112
T	116	/	112	/	97	111
W	108	/	108	/	99	107
T	113	/	111	/	91	99
F	102	/	91	/	91	101
S	108	/	102	/	99	98
S	96	/	94	/	95	97

Home Blood Sugar Reading – Week of Feb 24th - Mar 2nd 2003

	Reading Before Breakfast		Reading Before Lunch		Reading Before Dinner	Reading At Bedtime
M	99	/	106	/	85	91
T	100	/	106	/	95	91
W	96	/	102	/	96	95
T	103	/	102	/	92	98
F	107	/	109	/	101	99
S	107	/	103	/	100	98
S	105	/	106	/	100	109

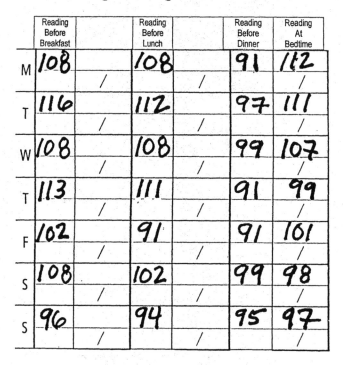

36

Home Blood Sugar Reading – Week of Mar 3rd - 9th 2003

	Reading Before Breakfast		Reading Before Lunch		Reading Before Dinner	Reading At Bedtime
M	119	/	109	/	110	109 /
T	112	/	111	/	110	115 /
W	119	/	99	/	98	100 /
T	108	/	109	/	96	98 /
F	102	/	97	/	93	95 /
S	96	/	101	/	100	101 /
S	95	/	103	/	103	109 /

Home Blood Sugar Reading – Week of Mar 10th – 16th 2003

	Reading Before Breakfast		Reading Before Lunch		Reading Before Dinner	Reading At Bedtime
M	117	/	117	/	101	108 /
T	104	/	107	/	104	95 /
W	95	/	97	/	90	99 /
T	95	/	102	/	92	96 /
F	102	/	103	/	101	99 /
S	107	/	99	/	93	97 /
S	99	/	97	/	92	97 /

Home Blood Sugar Reading – Week of Mar 17th – 23rd 2003

	Reading Before Breakfast		Reading Before Lunch		Reading Before Dinner	Reading At Bedtime
M	103	/	96	/	93	92
						/
T	91	/	97	/	88	85
						/
W	97	/	96	/	90	93
						/
T	92	/	90	/	90	93
						/
F	95	/	97	/	86	97
						/
S	97	/	96	/	96	95
						/
S	98	/	97	/	97	95
						/

There are several ways of testing blood sugar levels. One method is the "at home method" which I used and recorded in my personal records as you have just reviewed. There are also ways of testing your blood sugar at your physician's office. Please note that when I was attempting to refocus my life to come up with a method for reducing my blood sugars, cholesterol and weight levels, I did not operate without medical advice. During the entire time I was developing my own eating habits and other health programs I was being examined regularly by two physicians located in two different medical offices. Getting a "second opinion" is generally good advice, especially when one is facing a "life threatening disease". I did my home monitoring, as you have just seen, but I also wanted my physicians to examine my blood sugar and cholesterol levels to tell me what their medical tests indicated. Therefore, I had my doctors perform tests to determine my blood sugar and cholesterol levels on a monthly basis. This gave me medical numbers to compare with my home test numbers. The blood sugar tests performed on me by my physicians are known as "hemoglobin A1c tests".

Hemoglobin A1c tests

The medical books tell us that a hemoglobin A1c test is a type of blood test performed on people who are interested in knowing how much sugar is in their blood stream during a particular period of time. It is said that Hemoglobin A1c is a chemical combination of hemoglobin and glucose. The name hemoglobin refers to the part of the red blood cell that carries oxygen around in one's body. Glucose is another name for a type of sugars that circulate in a human's blood stream. The reason for taking the hemoglobin A1c test is that this medical blood test will tell a person how well blood is being controlled over an approximate three-month period of time. Two main reasons for taking a hemoglobin A1c test are (a) the test offers a 'second opinion' to confirm home blood sugar monitoring results and (b) it is written in the medical literature that there appears to be a direct relationship between hemoglobin A1c levels and the risk of life threatening diabetic disease problems. In simple language, the medical literature tells us that the higher the hemoglobin A1c level the greater the risk of developing coronary artery disease, blindness, kidney disease, neuropathy and possible partial or complete limb amputations.

Red blood cells in a person's body live about 90-120 days and old red blood cells are continually replaced by new red blood cells. As new red blood cells are created, circulating sugars in one's blood combine with hemoglobin to form hemoglobin

A1c. If one has a high level of sugar in the blood stream, the medical reports tell us that the A1c test will reflect this. If the level of sugar is within normal ranges, the A1c test will reflect that. If a person is reducing the level of blood sugar in his or her body, sequential Hemoglobin A1c test results may be represented on a piece of paper by a declining graph. If a person is not reducing the level of blood sugar in his or her blood stream, sequential test results may be represented by a steady or advancing graph. Each individual Hemoglobin A1c test result reflects the average sugar concentration in one's body over an approximate three-month period of time.

The numbers that the lab people and the medical people use when examining Hemoglobin A1c tests are these,

1. 4% to 6% is considered normal.
2. 7% or less is considered excellent blood sugar control for diabetics.
3. 7.1% to 8.0% is considered good blood sugar control for diabetics.
4. 8.1% to 9.0% is considered fair blood sugar control for diabetics.
5. 9.1% or higher is considered poor blood sugar control for diabetics.

On January 22, 2003, I had a hemoglobin A1c test performed on my blood and it came up 12.0%. Three points above the "poor blood sugar control level" listed above. Translating 12.0% to mg/dl levels, a 12.0% A1c Hemoglobin level generally equals a 300mg/dl level on a home or physician's monitor.

Was I scared when I learned that I had a blood sugar reading of 300 mg/dl and type 2 diabetes and that I had probably suffered unknowingly from this disease of diabetes for the previous seven years? **You bet I was scared. I was really scared.** Type 2 diabetes is a "life threatening" disease. It is something a person can, and should be, really scared about.

As indicated, after my first medical hemoglobin A1c test, I had my physicians perform several more A1c blood tests on me to determine my blood sugar levels on February 27th, March 27th, and April 30th and May 27th of 2003. With the new "one-step" food schedule I had adopted, I wanted to see if my home blood sugar monitoring results were being confirmed by medical Hemoglobin A1c tests.

When these four tests results, each approximately one month apart, were graphed, here is what the graph showed, (see next page).

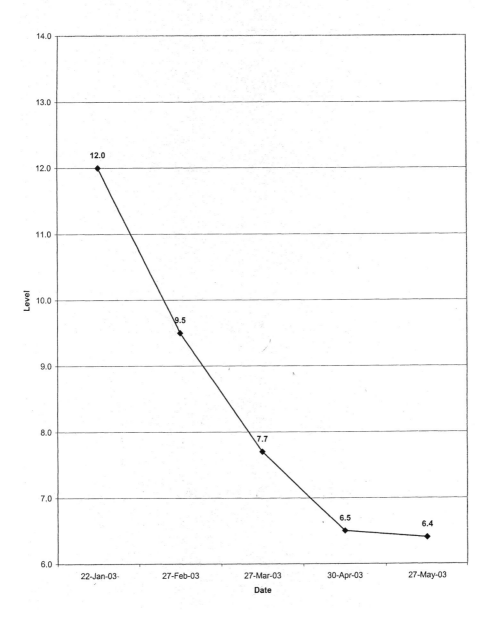

43

Remember that 7% or less is considered excellent blood sugar control for diabetics. My Hemoglobin test results performed at my physician's office, showed a decline from 12.0% to 6.4% in a very short period of time.

I had gone from "terrible or dangerous" blood sugar control to "excellent" blood sugar control in the time frame from January to April-May, 2003, **primarily due, in my opinion, from changing my food eating habits**. (Switching from List "B" foods to List "A" foods).

Since I had reduced my Hemoglobin A1c test results to a graph format, I then decided to do the same for my 2003 home monitor blood sugars test results. I used a weekly average for my home blood sugar results. The graph on the next page illustrates what my blood sugar levels looked like on my home monitor.

Blood Sugar - 15 Year Statistics
April 1988 - May 2003

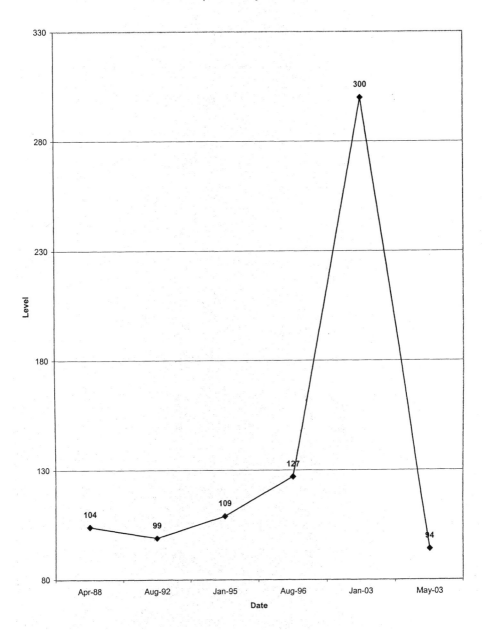

45

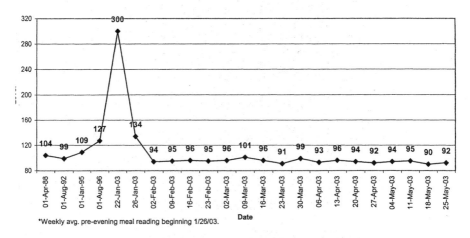

Blood Sugar - Weekly Average*
January 26 - May 25, 2003

*Weekly avg. pre-evening meal reading beginning 1/26/03.

While my physician was giving me my hemoglobin A1c blood sugar tests, he also measured my levels of cholesterol, my levels of HDL cholesterol, my levels of LDL cholesterol and my triglycerides levels. I took these numbers and graphed them as comparison with the numbers I had in my medical file dating pre-2003. Here then is my medical history pre-2003 and early 2003 as best reflected in these graphs,

Total Cholesterol - 15 Year Statistics
April 1988 - May 2003

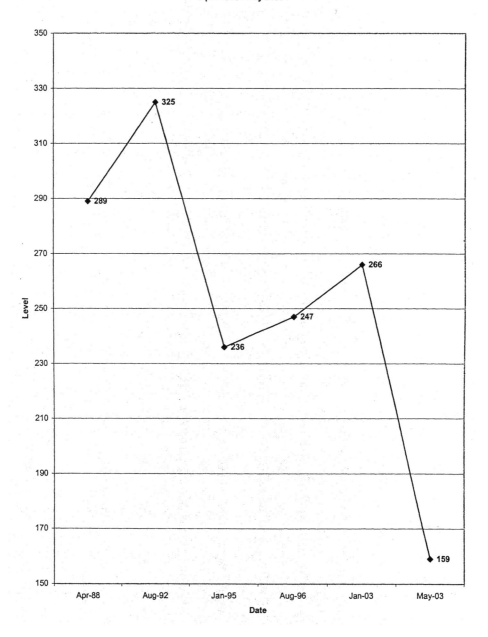

47

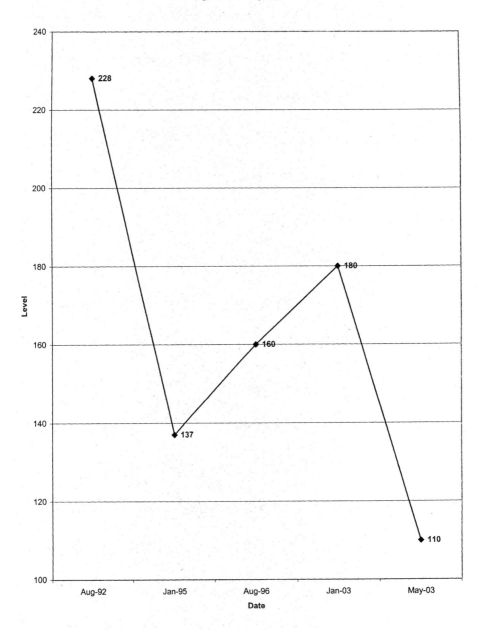

Cholesterol - LDL - 11 Year Statistics
August 1992 - May 2003

Cholesterol - HDL - 11 Year Statistics
August 1992 - May 2003

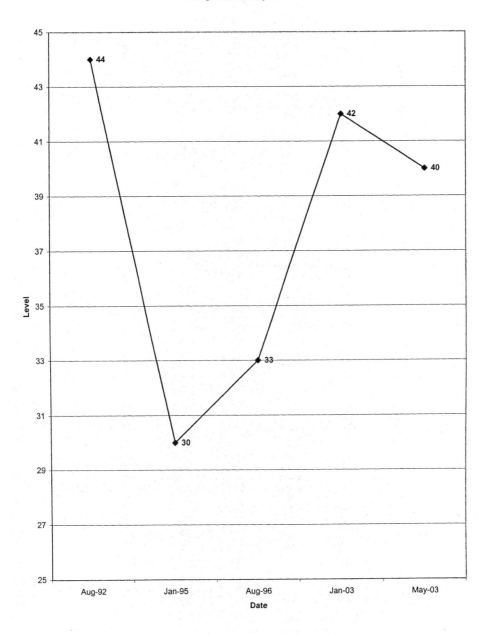

Triglycerides - 11 Year Statistics
August 1992 - May 2003

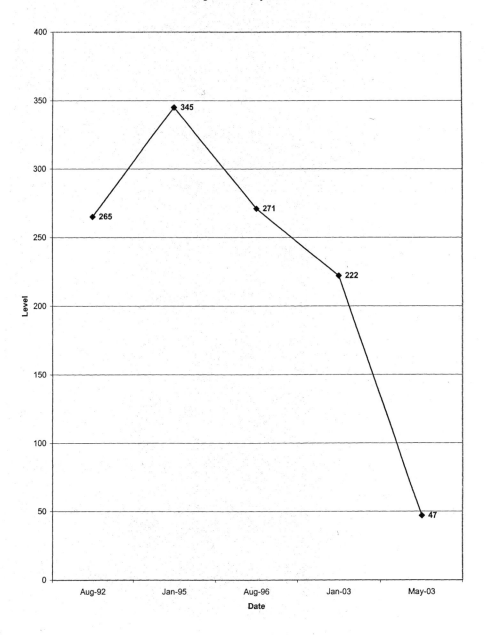

The medical literature seems to indicate that the various goals for cholesterols and triglycerides in one's body should be as follows:

Total cholesterol –a goal is a number less than 200.
HDL cholesterol – a goal is a number greater than 35.
LDL cholesterol – a goal is a number less than 100.
Triglycerides – a goal is a number less than 200.

These numbers are not fixed in concrete, different medical books give slightly different numbers, but the above table is fairly representative of the various goals for each category.

It is also possible to calculate cholesterol ratios. The medical literature tells a reader that the ratio of total cholesterol to HDL cholesterol is worth looking at and the ratio of LDL cholesterol to HDL cholesterol is also worth one's consideration. With this in mind, I graphed the ratio of my HDL, LDL and my total cholesterol levels.

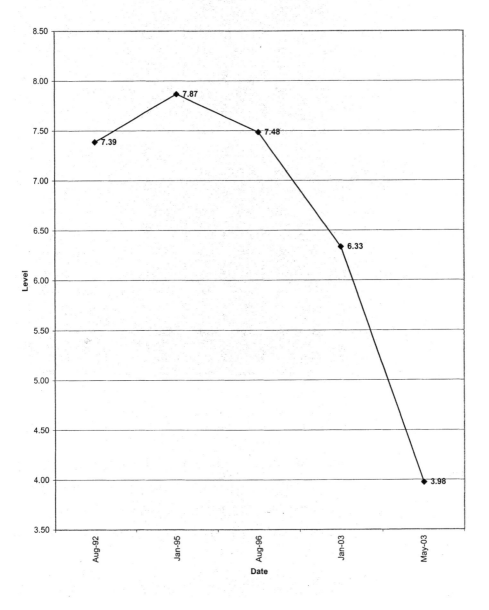

Total Cholesterol / HDL Ratio
Low Risk 3.3 - 4.4
Average Risk 4.4 - 7.1
Moderate Risk 7.1 - 11.0
High Risk 11.0+

52

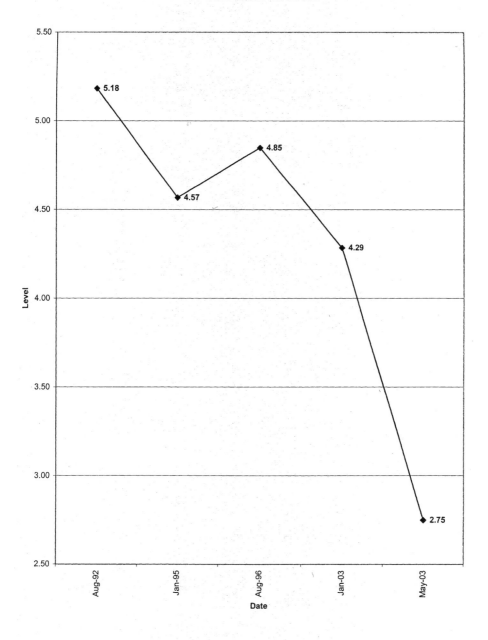

53

Blood Sugar Readings*

*Weekly avg. pre-evening meal reading beginning 1/26/03.

Week Ending:

01-Apr-88	**104**
01-Aug-92	**99**
01-Jan-95	**109**
01-Aug-96	**127**
22-Jan-03	**300**
26-Jan-03	**134**
02-Feb-03	**94**
09-Feb-03	**95**
16-Feb-03	**96**
23-Feb-03	**95**
02-Mar-03	**96**
09-Mar-03	**101**
16-Mar-03	**96**
23-Mar-03	**91**
30-Mar-03	**99**
06-Apr-03	**93**
13-Apr-03	**96**
20-Apr-03	**94**
27-Apr-03	**92**
04-May-03	**94**
11-May-03	**95**
18-May-03	**90**
25-May-03	**92**

Hemoglobin A1c

Blood Sugar Test Results

Date:

22-Jan-03	**12.0**
27-Feb-03	**9.5**
27-Mar-03	**7.7**
30-Apr-03	**6.5**
27-May-03	**6.4**

Tables giving raw numbers on which the above graphs are based.

Cholesterol LDL / HDL Ratio

The lower the number the less the risk.

Date:	LDL	HDL	LDL / HDL Ratio
Aug-92	228	44	5.18
Jan-95	137	30	4.57
Aug-96	160	33	4.85
Jan-03	180	42	4.29
May-03	110	40	2.75

Total Cholesterol / HDL Ratio

Low Risk	3.3 - 4.4
Average Risk	4.4 - 7.1
Moderate Risk	7.1 - 11.0
High Risk	11.0+

Date:	Total Cholesterol	HDL	Total Cholesterol / HDL Ratio
Aug-92	325	44	7.39
Jan-95	236	30	7.87
Aug-96	247	33	7.48
Jan-03	266	42	6.33
May-03	159	40	3.98

The Role of Exercise

I have never been much of a fan of exercise, perhaps I should have been. Prior to January 22nd, 2003, when I received the wake-up call that I was a full-fledged type 2 diabetic, I did very little exercise. Once I discovered my diabetic disease, however, I also discovered the benefits of exercise. It seems that exercise is good for diabetics, as it is for people who are overweight and people in general. My primary exercises now consists of walking from my office to my home and back again, once a day, plus a half-hour workout now and then on an exercise machine.

The walk to my home and back to my office appears to be beneficial, especially because my home is at the top of a rather high hill so that the walk up is always challenging, the walk back to the office a little easier.

When I was a younger person, I used to do "jumping jacks" and "sit-ups". I am still good for 50-100 sit-ups a day, but not too good for "jumping-jacks". Whatever exercise one undertakes, the literature seems to indicate that some exercise is very good for overweight persons and diabetics; either diagnosed diabetics or undiagnosed diabetics. I now utilize a program of exercise regularly and consider it an essential part of my health treatment program.

The Importance of Vitamins for me

Since the list of foods I now eat is a shorter list than the list of foods I used to eat, I did not want to find that my nutrient intake was lessened by my current food schedule. So I looked into vitamins. There are many books on vitamins and many food supplements that one can take to help improve health. The many vitamins I personally examined were these,

        One Source Multi
        Basic Anti-Ox Multi
        Calcium, Magnesium & Zinc Multi
        Fish Oil
        Flaxseed Oil
        Leutin
        Lycopene
        Mega-Pantethine
        Milk Thistle
        Pantothenic Acid (Vitamin B-5)
        Quercetin
        Selenium
        Super GLA
        Vitamin B-1
        Taurine
        Alpha Lipoic Acid
        Aspara-Plus

Beta Carotene
B Complex Vitamins Multi
Chromium Picolinate
Coenzyme Q-10
Garlic
Ginkgo Biloba
L-Carnitine
Saw Pelmetto
Vitamin B-3 (Niacin)
Biotin
Vitamin B-6 (Pyridoxine hydrochoride)
Vitamin B-12
Vitamin E
Folic Acid
Vitamin C
Plus a few others

Let's start off by saying that I am not an authority on vitamins. I am not even very knowledgeable about vitamins. I do not personally recommend that anyone take vitamins. On the other hand, I do not personally recommend that anyone not take vitamins. The issue of supplements seems to me to be an issue that each person must research and decide upon based on his or her own independent analysis, reading skills and advise from a medical doctor or health care provider.

The best way for anyone interested in the issue of vitamins is to arrive at his or her own decision by reviewing the literature located at a library, a health food store, or even on the internet plus consultation with a medical physician. Such literature and advice will give suggestions for nutrients, discuss which vitamins are said to be helpful for people in general, for people with diabetes, for people with high levels of cholesterol, for overweight people who decide to reduce their food intake, for people with neuropathy, for people with a lack of energy. Before beginning a vitamin program, get yourself educated is the best recommendation I can make and education normally begins by reading good books, good literature and talking with a professional in this field. If you do decide to research the issue of vitamins, the above list might be a good starting point for you to seek more knowledge about. What do these vitamins do for you, who recommends them, what are their benefits? Answers to these questions can be found in every good vitamin or supplement book (see appendix) and by talking to your doctor.

My personal experience with medicine

When I was told on January 22nd, 2003, that I had type 2 diabetes, I was almost floored. **It was the most devastating health news that I had ever received in my entire lifetime.** When I was further informed that my blood sugar levels should be around 90-110 mg/dl and they were at 300 mg/dl, I started to panic. I could see myself on the road to physical disaster or death. January 22nd, 2003, marks the biggest medical shock I have ever received in my lifetime and I hope never to receive such a shock again. I knew then that something had to be done and it has to be done **immediately** in order to preserve what little health I had left. In order to save my life, I personally undertook the following three steps,

1. I rejected the use of insulin for my type 2 diabetes because I was told that my disease was such that I probably did not immediately need to take insulin to stay alive. Had I been diagnosed with juvenile diabetes or had I been told that I had to take insulin or die, I would have certainly taken insulin.
2. I accepted the idea of an immediate use of a pharmaceutical drug to help me start reducing

the circulating sugars in my blood stream and to get me on the right track.

3. I immediately started to learn everything I could about type 2 diabetes and, within one day, I started to make changes in the foods I ate and the foods that I did not eat.

For me, the use of a pharmaceutical medicine was almost required. Remember on January 22, 2003, I knew almost nothing about type 2 diabetes. So, knowing almost nothing about type 2 diabetes, I signed up to take one pharmaceutical pill daily, hoping that I was not taking another Rezulin type drug. I took this drug for approximately 30 days during which time I carefully monitored my blood sugars daily. At the end of 30 days, I was having such success in lowering my blood sugars through the change in my food eating habits, my exercise program and the use of some of the vitamins listed in the previous table that I decided to go off the pharmaceutical drug. Remember, that two medical physicians, both of whom I eventually told that I had discontinued the use of the pharmaceutical drug, were monitoring my blood sugars carefully. **I would never recommend that anyone reduce or eliminate the use of any pharmaceutical drug without fully informing their physician and seeking the physician's advice before doing so.**

For myself, I then monitored my blood sugars even more carefully. I wanted to see if ending the drug would result in a higher daily or higher hourly blood sugar level. It did not seem to do so. My blood sugar levels had been so significantly reduced through my new food eating habits combined with my exercise and vitamin use program that the daily taking or the non-taking of one single tablet of a pharmaceutical drug which I had only been taking for about 30 days did not seem to make any difference. As I was only using a small quantity of the pharmaceutical drug, since I had only taken it for a very short period of time, and since the non-use of it did not seem to increase my blood sugar levels, I ended the use of this drug and have never taken it again. Thus within approximately 30 days of my being diagnosed as a type 2 diabetic, I was handling my disease with a food, exercise and a vitamin program and I was entirely insulin free and pharmaceutical drug free. **<u>Not only was I insulin free and drug free, but my blood sugar and my cholesterol levels were the best I had achieved in years.</u>**

In the next graph, you can see my blood sugar levels from January 22nd until May of 2003 based on my home blood sugar monitoring. I started taking the pharmaceutical medicine on January 24th,

2003 and I stopped taking this drug by the end of February 2003. As you can see from this graph, my blood sugar levels did not rise after I stopped taking the pharmaceutical drug on February 28th.

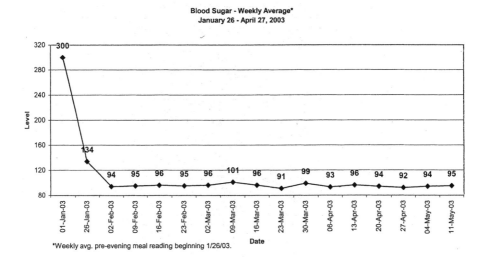

Blood Sugar - Weekly Average*
January 26 - April 27, 2003

*Weekly avg. pre-evening meal reading beginning 1/26/03.

What do all these graphs mean?

I prepared these graphs for myself and for my two physicians. I wanted to see what I could do to return myself to a healthy state. The graphs were simply an easy way to visualize what I accomplished within a 30-90 day period of time. The graphs told my two physicians and me that,

1. Within approximately 30 days of my being diagnosed as a type 2 diabetic, I had lowered my blood sugar levels to the levels that existed prior to 1996.
2. Within approximately 90 days of my being diagnosed as a type 2 diabetic, I had lowered my cholesterol levels to a 15-year low.
3. Within approximately 90 days of my being diagnosed as a type 2 diabetic, I had lowered my LDL cholesterol levels to an 11-year low.
4. Within approximately 90 days of my being diagnosed as a type 2 diabetic, I had lowered my triglycerides level to an 11-year low.
5. Within approximately 90 days of my being diagnosed as a type 2 diabetic I had lowered my total cholesterol/HDL ratio to an 11-year low.
6. Within approximately 90 days of my being diagnosed as a type 2 diabetic I had lowered my LDL/HDL cholesterol ratio to an 11-year low.

While my blood sugar levels had now returned to normal, **in less than 90 days my cholesterol, my LDL and my triglycerides levels were, most likely, at levels not seen, in my lifetime, for 20-30 years.** This is just a guess, but I would doubt that I ever had such low cholesterol, LDL, triglyceride and ratio levels in my entire adult lifetime. The reason that my graphs reflect only 15-year lows and 11-year lows is because this is as far back as the medical records at my physician's office went. My physician had no medical records for me beyond 15 years. He did not have HDL, LDL, or triglyceride levels for me beyond 11 years. But if I had a complete medical printout from the time I was a teenager, I would bet that the results achieved in the 90 days of early 2003 would have broken records for as far back as my adult life existed.

And I felt wonderful. In every aspect of my body I felt better. No longer was I tired, urinating all the time, thirsty, dehydrated with pressure building up behind my eyes. **I felt wonderful.** If there were "10" ways to rank how one feels with respect to one's body, I would rank my feeling on January 22nd, of 2003, at about a "3" and my feeling in May, of 2003, as a "10". **I felt absolutely great; the change in less than 90 days was unbelievable.**

My approach consisted of primarily selecting the foods I was eating from the list I have given you. This list is not a static list. It is not fixed in concrete. I add to it all the time. If I find something that tastes good or is good for me and does not have a lot of carbohydrates in it, I add this food to my list. The list grows day by day as I discover new foods to eat that do not keep my blood sugar levels high. I try to reduce my intake of carbohydrates and having a list of acceptable foods to eat makes this task easy to do. I don't count the carbohydrates I eat at each meal, I just try to eat no more than I can consume while maintaining my blood sugar levels around the 90 mg/dl-110 mg/dl pre-meal levels. If I started to see higher fasting or pre-meal blood sugar numbers than that, I would start to immediately reduce my daily carbohydrate intake.

It is my personal opinion that the key to my personal health recovery program is a drastic reduction in the amount of carbohydrates I eat on a daily basis as compared to the quantity of carbohydrates that I was eating in the seven years from 1996-January 22, 2003. **The food program I was following from 1996-2003 was on its way to killing me. I believe that the food program I am now on will add years to my life**.

As indicated, I also take vitamins from those on the list provided, and I try to exercise regularly. **I rank my eating habits as of primary importance.** I consider my exercise program as having secondary importance and my vitamin use as thirdly important.

I believe it has been the change in my food habits that has been 95% responsible for the drastic improvement in my blood sugar levels, my total cholesterol levels, my HDL, LDL, and triglyceride levels and the general overall improvement of my health.

Weight Control

The primary reason I adopted my approach of food-exercise-vitamins to my health needs was to avoid the harmful consequences of type 2 diabetes. I did not select this approach in order to lose weight. However, the loss of weight seemed to come natural with this method of eating, exercising and using vitamins. At my peak in the late 90's, I weighed 205 pounds. By April of 2003, I was settled in at a comfortable 175 pounds. The total loss of 30 pounds did not occur because of my new program. I had already lost considerable weight by January 22nd, 2003, as my body was "wasting away" by my type 2 diabetes, "the wasting disease". However, when I started eating fewer carbohydrates, exercising and taking vitamins on a daily basis, what excess body weight I still had seemed to go away almost without effort. 175 pounds is a very comfortable weight for me, I am

5 foot 10 inches tall, and I feel light on my feet, quick in my step and full of great energy at my current weight and blood sugar levels. I had not weighed 175 pounds since high school and carrying a load 30 pounds lighter than my peak weight is a very pleasant situation to be in.

As I indicated before, and I wish to repeat it here, I personally believe that I would never have developed the disease of type 2 "diabetes" if I had not been significantly overweight and eating too many carbohydrates in the seven-year period from 1996 until January 22, 2003.

<u>I am 100% convinced that my disease of diabetes was a direct result of,</u>

1. Being overweight, and
2. Eating too many carbohydrates for those seven years.

The Dangers Associated with the disease "diabetes".

It has been written that the number of people who have type 2 diabetes is increasing so rapidly that it will soon be a global epidemic. Today in the United States more than 16,000,000 people have diabetes. It is estimated that 1 in 3 children born in the year 2000 will suffer from the disease of diabetes before their life is over. It is reported that millions of people have diabetes today without even knowing it. You may be one of those people. Remember, I had diabetes for seven long years and did not discover this fact until January of 2003. The chance of an overweight adult in America having "undiagnosed diabetes" today is very high. Any adult who has the symptoms of this disease should seek a blood sugar test from his or her physician to establish the mg/dl blood sugar levels in his or her body in order to discover whether or not such an individual also suffers from "undiagnosed" diabetes, just as I did.

To repeat what I have said before, diabetes is not a mild benign disease. The medical literature tells us that **diabetes is a serious life-threatening disease**. Diabetes carries with it many risks including,

1. The risk of kidney damage.
2. The risk of coronary heart disease.
3. The risk of blindness.
4. The risk of liver damage.
5. The risk of neuropathy.
6. The risk of limb amputation.
7. The risk of general damage to one's health.

All people with diabetes have one thing in common. They have too much sugar or glucose circulating in their blood. Most people with type 2 diabetes have other things in common also, they are often thirsty, they are often tired, they frequently have to urinate, they have blurred vision, their skin may feel dry which is caused by the dehydration going on in their bodies, they may feel pain in their legs. People with type 2 diabetes generally feel lousy and tired much of the time. **<u>In addition many type 2 diabetics are overweight</u>**. Each day 1,800 new cases of diabetes are diagnosed in the United States, over 600,000 new cases each year. Over ninety percent of the people who are over 20 years of age and who have diabetes have type 2 diabetes. Type 1 diabetes, often called juvenile diabetes, is generally found in younger people and often involves a total inability to produce insulin. Most type 2 diabetics still produce insulin in their pancreas. The medical literature tells us that the problem type 2 diabetics often have is a resistance problem whereby the sugars that are cir-culating in their bodies are, for one reason or anoth-er or for reasons unknown, not able to enter individ-ual cells in a normal non-diabetic fashion. This may be known as "resistance" in some of the literature you may read. What happens, in effect, is that the blood sugars in a type 2 diabetic's body are not being used efficiently by that person's blood cells and so they are urinated away in the devastating "wasting disease" known as type 2 diabetes.

The most important thing for an overweight non-diabetic person is not to get diabetes in the first place. Avoiding the disease is the best pos-sible solution to solving the problems of the dis-ease. In general, the medical literature tells us that once a person has type 2 diabetes that person must either adopt some method to control this disease or that person should be prepared to live a life aware of the risks associated with diabetes. For myself, when I was diagnosed as a "type 2 diabetic", it did not take me long to realize that if I continued with blood sugar levels at 300mg/dl I was a walking dead-man. I wanted to have a life. I didn't want to face,

1. The **required use** of insulin, or
2. The **required use** of pharmaceutical drugs.

And so, virtually overnight, I set out to learn as much as I could about my disease. Learning as much as I could I, **almost immediately, changed my food habits** and began a program of exercise and vitamin consumption. The result of this effort to save my life by **changing my food consumption habits** was that within approximately 90 days, in less than 30 days in some cases,

1. My **blood sugar** returned to below my pre-diabetic levels.
2. My **cholesterol was at a 15 year low**. (Possibly a 20-30 year low)
3. My **LDL was at an 11 year low**. (Possibly a 20-30 year low)
4. My **HDL was above 35**. (Which was my goal)
5. My **triglycerides were at an 11 year low**, (Possibly at an all-lifetime low)
6. My weight was at a comfortable 175 pounds, and,
7. **I felt better than I had felt in years**, I was a "10" on a scale of "1-10" and I began to feel wonderful again.

Will my approach of reduced carbohydrate intake, along with a little exercise and some vitamin intake work for you? **I don't know what will work for you or for anyone else. I know only what, in less than 90 days, worked for me.**

This much I will tell you, if you are concerned about excess weight, if you are concerned about your high cholesterol levels, if you are concerned about your high triglyceride levels, **do not switch to the food program that I selected for myself without first talking with your doctor.**

Your doctor is the person best able to advise you if such a food program might be useful for you. I am not a physician and I know nothing about medicine. I only know what worked for my cholesterol levels, my LDL cholesterol levels, my triglycerides levels, blood sugar levels, my weight and me to control my type 2 diabetes. The method outlined in this report should not be tried by you without first completely discussing such a method with your physician and only taking such action or non-action as your physician advises you.

I am not a medical doctor and I do not give medical advice and I am not telling you what to do or what not to do. If you are overweight and have high cholesterol levels or already have some of the consequences of diabetes such as kidney disease,

liver disease, coronary artery disease, neuropathy, eye disease or nerve disease, the approach that worked for me may not work for you. By all means do nothing without your doctor's complete knowledge, advice, and recommendation.

This report is just one man's story, a historically accurate record of what worked for one man and how he was able to control his weight, cholesterol levels, triglyceride levels, blood sugar levels and his type 2 diabetes" without,

1. A life-long commitment to insulin, and without
2. A life-long commitment to pharmaceutical drugs.

It is estimated that 140 million people worldwide have the disease of diabetes and it is reported that this number will double by the year 2025. It is written that in the country of India alone, 30 million people are "diabetic". Millions of overweight people are said to have the disease of "diabetes" without even knowing it. This is why "diabetes" is said to be **"the silent killer"**.

The name for this disease is "diabetes mellitus". The name comes a combination of a Greek word meaning "to siphon" and a Latin word meaning "sweet like honey". The high level of sugar in one's urine is what gives diabetes its name. Diabetes is also known as the "wasting disease" because a person's life seems to be "wasting away" as sugars and nutrients are steadily "urinated away".

In the very old days, before modern science, it has been written that one means of testing for diabetes was to place one's urine by insects that feed on sugar. If the insects came to the urine, the patient was "diabetic". What is the cause of type 1 and type 2 "diabetes"? No one absolutely knows for sure, but there are some general thoughts about the factors that might be associated with the contracting of this disease. One factor is **heredity**. Another factor may be **excess body weight**. Another factor may be the consumption of **junk foods and foods containing high carbohydrate and sugar levels**.

Schools, hospitals, cafeterias, many quick-stop restaurants often serve food high in simple sugars and carbohydrates. It seems common sense that the more sugar one eats, the more sugar in the blood stream. Drink a lot of alcohol and you will find lots of alcohol in your blood stream. The police even have portable monitors for measuring exactly how much alcohol is in anyone's blood at any particular time. Most likely the same scenario applies to sugar and carbohydrates. Consume a lot of carbohydrates and sugars and you will find a lot of sugar in your blood stream. The exact amount can be established by the blood tests at a physician's office or by using a home blood sugar monitoring device.

Because diabetes is such a deadly disease, any person with diabetes should be under the care of a family physician or medical team. It is not advisable to try to control one's diabetes without the help of the medical profession. When I was told that I had type 2 diabetes, I consulted two physicians and worked out my food-exercise-and vitamin program while seeing these two physicians on a regular basis.

As I said before, it is my personal opinion that had I used my current food program in 1996 to control my weight and carbohydrate intake during the seven years from 1996 to 2003, I do not believe I would have ever contracted the disease of "diabetes" in the first place. I personally believe I became a diabetic primarily by not controlling my,

1. **Weight, and**
2. **Carbohydrate intake.**

Once I stopped eating so much carbohydrate, and got my weight under control, my cholesterol dropped, my LDL dropped, my blood sugar levels dropped and my triglyceride levels dropped, my cholesterol/HDL ratio improved, my LDL/HDL ratio improved.

For me, it seemed almost a miracle. All this happened in less than 90 days and my blood sugars were back to pre-1996 levels in less than 30 days. Today, I

1. Generally eat the low carbohydrate foods listed in list "A", pages 25-26.
2. Generally don't eat the high carbohydrate foods listed in list "B", pages 27-28.
3. Engage in some exercise.
4. Take some vitamins.
5. Use no pharmaceutical drugs of any kind.
6. Take no insulin injections of any kind.

My energy level has returned, I no longer feel tired all the time, I don't urinate as often during the day or evening hours, the pressure on my eyes has greatly diminished and I don't feel I face the risk of limb amputation. I have been medically tested for kidney and liver problems and show no sign of either. I am still a "type 2 diabetic" but you would never know it if you passed me on the street. I look no different than any average person my age who is non-diabetic.

If you have fears of excess weight, if you have high cholesterol levels, if you are worried about the possibility of yourself or someone you love becoming diabetic in the future or, if you have any of the symptoms listed below,

1. A frequent desire to urinate.
2. An unusual thirst.
3. Blurred vision.
4. A feeling of being tired most of the time for no apparent reason.
5. Leg pain
6. Nerve damage
7. Poor circulation.

Then you may want to study my charts and graphs as presented in this report and talk them over with your family physician. Following not mine, for I am not giving you any medical advice, but following only your own doctor's medical advice you may wish to test out a similar (a) food (b) exercise and (c) vitamin program for yourself. It just possible that what worked for me, might also work for you. Or might also work for someone you love.

To repeat what I am now saying for a third time, had I known in 1996 what I know today, I do not believe I would ever have become a "diabetic" in the first place. I believe my disease of diabetes was brought on by solely by my (a) excess weight and (b) excess consumption of carbohydrates.

If you or someone you love has an excess weight problem or a high cholesterol problem and think you are consuming too many carbohydrates, **then TALK TO YOUR DOCTOR.**

If your doctor agrees, get yourself a good home blood sugar monitor and start having regular medical checkups. Compare your blood sugar, cholesterol, HDL, LDL, triglyceride and HDL/LDL/cholesterol ratio numbers with mine. Check the results achieved by your food-exercise-vitamin program to see if what worked so well for me might also work equally as well for you.

I call my method the "one-step method" because all it took for me was "one-step" to put this method into practice. I took the one-step of going from a life-style of eating high carbohydrate list "B" foods to a new life-style of eating low carbohydrate list "A" foods. I attribute 95% of my good blood sugar, HDL, LDL, total cholesterol and triglyceride test results to the fact that I am now eating the foods that I have listed for you. Just one-step was all it took for me to return my health test results to record levels.

1. **If you have a high cholesterol level,** discuss my list "A" and list "B" with your physician to see if your physician recommends that you make the "one-step" switch from eating only foods in list "B" to eating only foods in list "A". Ask your doctor if such a "one-step" switch will substantially lower your cholesterol levels as such a "one-step" switch lowered my cholesterol levels.

2. **If you are substantially overweight,** discuss my list "A" and list "B" with your physician to see if your physician recommends that you make the "one-step" switch from eating only foods in list "B" to eating only foods in list "A". Ask your doctor if such a "one-step" switch will substantially lower your weight levels as such a "one-step" switch lowered my weight levels.

3. **If you have low HDL cholesterol levels,** discuss my list "A" and list "B" with your physician to see if your physician recommends that you make the "one-step" switch from eating only foods in list "B" to eating only foods in list "A". Ask if your doctor if such a "one-step" switch will substantially raise your HDL cholesterol levels.

4. **If you have a high LDL cholesterol levels,** discuss my list "A" and list "B" with your

physician to see if your physician recommends that you make the "one-step" switch from eating only foods in list "B" to eating only foods in list "A". Ask your doctor if such a "one-step" switch will substantially lower your LDL cholesterol levels as such a "one-step" switch lowered my LDL cholesterol levels.

5. **If you have a high triglyceride levels,** discuss my list "A" and list "B" with your physician to see if your physician recommends that you make the "one-step" switch from eating only foods in list "B" to eating only foods in list "A". Ask your doctor if such a "one-step" switch will substantially lower your triglyceride levels as such a "one-step" switch lowered my triglyceride levels.

6. **If you have a poor HDL/LDL/total cholesterol ratios,** discuss my list "A" and list "B" with your physician to see if your physician recommends that you make the "one-step" switch from eating only foods in list "B" to eating only foods in list "A". Ask your doctor if such a "one-step" switch will substantially improve your HDL/LDL total cholesterol ratios as such a "one-step" switch improved my cholesterol ratios.

7. **If you have a high blood sugar levels,** discuss my list "A" and list "B" with your physician to

see if your physician recommends that you make the "one-step" switch from eating only foods in list "B" to eating only foods in list "A". Ask your doctor if such a "one-step" switch will substantially lower your blood sugar levels as such a "one-step" switch substantially lowered my blood sugar levels.

8. **If you do not yet have diabetes and are worried about possibly getting diabetes,** discuss my list "A" and list "B" with your physician to see if your physician recommends that you make the "one-step" switch from eating only foods in list "B" to eating only foods in list "A". Ask your doctor if such a "one-step" switch will substantially reduce your risk of ever getting diabetes in the first place.

If you ever, and only with the recommendation of your physician, take the same one-step from list "B" to list "A" that I took, I would hope that you are also able to lower your cholesterol, lower your weight, stabilize your blood sugar levels, raise your HDL, lower your LDL, increase your ratios, and improve your health test results just as I was able, by taking this simple "one-step", to improve mine. Good luck and best wishes!

Respectfully submitted,

—Bruce G. Gould

Once a diabetic, always a diabetic

If I were to walk into a physician's office today, a physician who had never treated me before, and if that physician were to put me through a series of medical tests, he would probably conclude that I was **not a diabetic.**

My fasting blood sugars would be between 90 and 110mg/dl. My cholesterol would be around 159, my HDL cholesterol about 40, my LDL cholesterol close to 110. My triglycerides should stay below 50. The ratio of my LDL to my HDL would be in the neighborhood of 2.75 and the ratio of my total cholesterol to my HDL cholesterol around 3.98.

This new physician would look at my test results and he or she might even say, "You are in great health, Bruce. The tests show you to have no major health problems". If I asked this new physician if the tests showed that I was a diabetic, the answer might be, "Of course not, to be a diabetic you need to have a fasting blood sugar level of 127mg/dl or above and your fasting blood sugar is 95". But, of course, I really am a diabetic, a diabetic with his blood sugar under control. If I were to start eating the foods I no longer eat and discontinue eating the foods I now eat, my blood sugar levels would, most likely, rise above 127. If I stopped my exercising and the use of vitamins, I might well be headed back up to the 300mg/dl blood sugar levels that I once reached. I am not fooling myself. Once a diabetic, always a diabetic and the only reason new medical tests today would show me as non-diabetic is because I have learned how to control my diabetes with a good food program, with exercise and with the use of vitamins.

My blood sugar problem is not solved; it is merely under control. That is okay with me. I would rather be a diabetic with his blood sugar under control than a diabetic with out of control blood sugar levels or a non-diagnosed diabetic who does not even know he is seriously ill with diabetes in the first place.

Once a diabetic, always a diabetic, the medical literature tells us. I can accept that. I am a diabetic with good blood sugar control. I can live with that.

There are numerous types of home blood sugar monitors. Any pharmacy will have several types. Two well-known types are listed below.

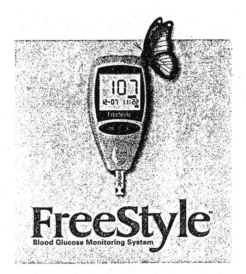

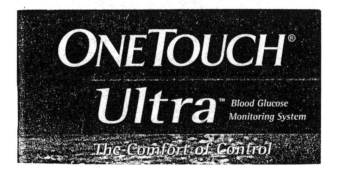

To ascertain how many carbohydrates are contained in any packaged food. Take total carbohydrates, deduct from that amount dietary fiber, multiply that amount by servings per container and you have a pretty good idea of the total carbohydrates or sugars within the package or can of food that you are examining. The amount varies considerably from food to food.

Nutrition Facts

Serving Size 2.5 oz. (70g/about 1/3 cup)(1cup prepared)
Servings Per Container about 3

Amount Per Serving	as packaged	as prepared†
Calories	250	390
Calories from Fat	10	150

	% Daily Value**

		% Daily Value**
Total Fat 1g*	2%	26%
Saturated Fat 0g	0%	51%
Cholesterol 0mg	0%	15%
Sodium 630mg	26%	32%
Total Carbohydrate 51g	17%	17%
Dietary Fiber 2g	8%	7%
Sugars 10g		
Protein 9g		

Vitamin A	0%	15%
Vitamin C	0%	0%
Calcium	6%	8%
Iron	10%	10%

* Amount as packaged
† Prepared as directed with butter and 2% milk.
** Percent Daily Values are based on a 2,000 calorie diet. Your daily values may be higher or lower depending on your calorie needs:

	Calories:	2,000	2,500
Total Fat	Less than	65g	80g
Sat. Fat	Less than	20g	25g
Cholest.	Less than	300mg	300mg
Sodium	Less than	2,400mg	2,400mg
Total Carb.		300g	375g
Dietary Fiber		25g	30g

Calories per gram:

Fat 9 • Carbohydrate 4 • Protein 4

Nutrition Facts

Serving Size 8 crackers (31g)
(1 serving = 2 full cracker sheets)
Servings Per Container About 13

Amount Per Serving

Calories 120   Calories from Fat 15

	% Daily Value*
Total Fat 1.5g	2%
Saturated Fat 0g	0%
Polyunsaturated Fat 0g	
Monounsaturated Fat 0g	
Cholesterol 0mg	0%
Sodium 190mg	8%
Total Carbohydrate 26g	9%
Dietary Fiber Less than 1g	3%
Sugars 8g	
Protein 2g	

Vitamin A 0%	•	Vitamin C 0%
Calcium 15%	•	Iron 6%

*Percent Daily Values are based on a 2,000 calorie diet. Your daily values may be higher or lower depending on your calorie needs:

	Calories:	2,000	2,500
Total Fat	Less than	65g	80g
Sat Fat	Less than	20g	25g
Cholesterol	Less than	300mg	300mg
Sodium	Less than	2,400mg	2,400mg
Total Carbohydrate		300g	375g
Dietary Fiber		25g	30g

→

Nutrition Facts
Serving Size 1 cup (245g)
Servings Per Container about 2

Amount Per Serving

Calories 10   Calories from Fat 5

	% Daily Value*
Total Fat 0.5g	1%
Saturated Fat 0g	0%
Cholesterol 0mg	0%
Sodium 970mg	40%
Total Carbohydrate 0g	0%
Sugars 0g	0%
Protein 1g	

Iron 6%

Not a significant source of dietary fiber, vitamin A, vitamin C and calcium.

* Percent Daily Values are based on a 2,000 calorie diet.

→

Nutrition Facts
Serving Size 1/2 cup (127g)
Servings Per Container 3

Amount Per Serving

Calories 30   Calories from Fat 0

	%Daily Value*
Total Fat 0g	0%
Saturated Fat 0g	0%
Cholesterol 0mg	0%
Sodium 440mg	18%
Potassium 410g	12%
Total Carbohydrate 4g	1%
Dietary Fiber 2g	8%
Sugars less than 1g	
Protein 3g	

Vitamin A 70% • Vitamin C 20%

Calcium 8% • Iron 15%

* Percent Daily Values are based on a 2,000 calorie diet.

→

Nutrition Facts
Serving Size 1 bar (28g)
Servings Per Container 10

Amount Per Serving

Calories 120   Calories from Fat 40

	% Daily Value*
Total Fat 4.5g	7%
Saturated Fat 1.5g	6%
Cholesterol 0mg	0%
Sodium 105mg	4%
Total Carbohydrate 19g	6%
Dietary Fiber 1g	5%
Sugars 8g	
Protein 3g	

Iron   2%

Not a significant source of Vitamin A, Vitamin C and Calcium.

→

Nutrition Facts
Serving Size 1 packet (20 g)
Servings Per Container 8

Amount Per Serving	One Packet	with 1 cup Fat Free Vit A & D Milk
Calories	70	150
Calories from Fat	5	10
	%Daily Value**	
Total Fat 0.5g*	1%	2%
Saturated Fat 0 g	0%	3%
Cholesterol <5 mg	1%	2%
Sodium 70 mg	3%	8%
Potassium 300 mg	9%	20%
Total Carbohydrate 12 g	4%	8%
Dietary Fiber <1 g	4%	4%
Sugars 7 g***		
Protein 4 g	9%	25%

87

There are many books on vitamins and supplements. A good starting point might be the book listed below. Other such books are available on the Internet or at your library.

<u>The Best Supplements for Your Health</u>, by Goldberg, Gitomer and Abel. Published by Twin Streams, Kensington Publishing Company, ISBN 0-7582-0219-9, Telephone 1-800-221-2647

Eggs and Cholesterol

When I decided to preserve what little health I had left by controlling my blood sugars through food, exercise and vitamins, I ran a test for myself on the issue of eating eggs.

There is much of nutritional value in an egg. On the other hand, many medical professionals, especially cardiologists, advise against eating too many eggs because eggs contain LDL cholesterol and excess LDL cholesterol levels are best avoided.

For my test, I had my LDL cholesterol levels checked at my physician's office when eggs were not in my diet. I then consumed about 2-6 eggs a day in the form of deviled eggs. I did this for about 30 days and had my LDL cholesterol levels measured again. I then stopped eating eggs altogether for 30 days and had my LDL cholesterol levels measured again. The result is a graph showing the effect that eating eggs seemed to have on my personal LDL cholesterol levels. If you would like a copy of this graph mail a self-addressed stamped envelope to: Bruce Gould, PO Box 1070, Okanogan, Washington, 98840 and request my "Egg and LDL Cholesterol study". I will send this study to you by return mail at no charge.

I don't expect to make any money.

I am not opening up my medical records and sharing my life experience as a diagnosed type 2 diabetic because I expect to make any money; this is not a moneymaking venture for me. I am sharing my experiences with you because I think it is the **right thing to do.**

My blood sugar is now under control. As I indicated, if I were to go to a new physician's office today and he or she was to give me a standard lipid and urine test it would undoubtedly show that I was not a diabetic and that I was in near perfect health. All my numbers would be within acceptable ranges. But you and I know better. I am not in perfect health, it just seems that way. I am still a diabetic; I am a diabetic who is as close to perfect health as he can probably get with his disease.

It is written that a good person should pass down to posterity his actions, his glory and successes; he should also pass on his understanding of the dangers, misfortunes, and mistakes in life. In this way, the first navigators of difficult waters marked the reefs they were able to avoid, and taught their successors how to navigate a safe route among the dangerous rocks. Nothing can make these reefs of life disappear but many can be approached or steered clear of, thanks to the teaching of experience by a good teacher and a good man.

I consider myself a good man and if I can help one person avoid the serious risks to health that come with the disease of diabetes my existence on this earth shall be more than justified

Changing my food habits, doing a little exercise, taking some vitamins is a program that helped to turn my life around. I now feel "10" on a scale of "1-10" and I take neither insulin nor drugs of any kind.

Do not, however, attempt the food, exercise and vitamin program that I am using without first discussing this with your doctor. Remember that during the entire time that I was developing my food-exercise-vitamin program I was continually seeing two physicians. Also remember that after I stopped using my pharmaceutical drug, I informed both my physicians that I had done the same. I viewed my physicians as two people who were there to help me and I made maximum use of their help as I struggled to save my life. Learning to develop a food-exercise-vitamin program does not mean leaving medical professionals out of the picture. If you adopt such a program, your decision gives you more reason to include a doctor in your activities, not less. It will be your doctor who will administer your medical tests and who will give you advice along the way as you attempt to avoid or control the disease of diabetes.

As I said at the beginning of this section, I am not opening up my medical records and sharing my experience with you as a diagnosed type 2 diabetic because I expect to make any money from this disclosure. This is not a moneymaking venture for me. I am sharing my experiences with you because I think it is the **right thing to do.** If I can help one person avoid the serious risks to health that come with the disease of diabetes my existence on this earth shall be more than justified

With best wishes, always,

—Bruce Gould